G000149796

Low Carb Cookbook

Quick, Easy, and Delicious Low Carb Recipes for Weight Loss

Amanda Hopkins

Text copyright © 2020 Amanda Hopkins - All Rights Reserved.

This document is geared towards providing exact and reliable information in regards to the topic and issue covered. The publication is sold with the idea that the publisher is not required to render accounting, officially permitted, or otherwise, qualified services. If advice is necessary, legal or professional, a practiced individual in the profession should be ordered.

From a Declaration of Principles which was accepted and approved equally by a Committee of the American Bar Association and a Committee of Publishers and Associations.

In no way is it legal to reproduce, duplicate, or transmit any part of this document in either electronic means or in printed format. Recording of this publication is strictly prohibited and any storage of this document is not allowed unless with written permission from the publisher. All rights reserved.

The information provided herein is stated to be truthful and consistent, in that any liability, in terms of inattention or otherwise, by any usage or abuse of any policies, processes, or directions contained within is the solitary and utter responsibility of the recipient reader. Under no circumstances will any legal responsibility or blame be held against the publisher for any reparation, damages, or monetary loss due to the information herein, either directly or indirectly.

Respective authors own all copyrights not held by the publisher.

The information herein is offered for informational purposes solely, and is universal as so. The presentation of the information is without contract or any type of guarantee assurance.

The trademarks that are used are without any consent, and the publication of the trademark is without permission or backing by the trademark owner. All trademarks and brands within this book are for clarifying purposes only and are owned by the owners themselves, not affiliated with this document.

ISBN: 978-1-64842-090-0

Table of Contents

Chapter 1: Introduction to The Low Carb Diet

Perhaps you've heard of the low carbohydrate or low carb diet, and wonder what the benefits are? In simple terms, this way of eating consists of restricting carbohydrates and increasing protein and fat. Two main benefits of eating this way are weight loss and feeling more energetic.

Many people struggle to lose weight and keep it off when following a low-fat high-carb diet because they often feel hungry. If you've ever been on such a dietary plan, you know the feeling of constantly being hungry. Not only that, but weight loss is often quite slow, which can lead to frustration and discouragement.

What is a Low Carb Diet?

A low carb diet does not mean cutting out all carbohydrates. This will not cause more weight loss, and in fact, it will hinder it. Normally, you should keep your carbohydrate intake to around 10–20 percent daily, especially in the beginning.

The low carb diet suggests that you eat fewer than 50 grams of carbs per day. There are some symptoms you may experience as your body adjusts to a new way of eating and burning energy. The symptoms include headaches, fatigue, flu-like feelings, weakness, and dizziness. These typically subside after a week or two of restricting carbs. After this phase, you will begin to experience increased energy, less hunger, and of course, weight loss.

What is Ketosis?

When you follow a low carb diet, your body enters a metabolic state known as ketosis. During this stage, the body becomes extremely efficient at burning fat to make energy and converts the fat in the liver into ketones. In this phase, you won't experience the blood sugar spikes that cause that sluggish feeling a couple of hours after eating a high-carb meal. It is also in this stage where weight loss happens more easily. Many people battling epilepsy and children who have suffered from prolonged and dangerous seizures, follow a ketosis diet because it improves their conditions.

Why Follow a Low Carb Diet?

The biggest reason people follow a low carbohydrate diet is to lose weight and keep the weight off. If you've struggled with yo-yo dieting, as many people have, restricting carbs is a great way to put an end to a vicious cycle.

Many diabetics follow a low carb eating plan for life because it keeps their blood glucose levels steady. It can help reduce or in some cases eliminate medications. Of course, if you are diabetic, you should always talk to your treating physician to see if restricting carbs would be beneficial for you.

If you are a big eater, you'll love the low-carb diet because you can eat quite a bit of food. However, in time, you'll find you'll eat less as your body adapts to the diet.

One of the greatest benefits to low-carb eating is never counting calories. If you've been a calorie-counter, this will be a welcome change for you. Restricting calories may cause weight loss, but you'll feel constantly hungry, which of course will eventually cause cheating or forfeiting the diet entirely. It can also lead to gaining the lost weight in addition to a few extra pounds.

What to Eat and What to Avoid on the Low Carb Diet

If you're considering trying the low carbohydrate diet, you may envision yourself eating large amounts of meat. But there are many other foods to choose from. In fact, making sure you eat plenty of vegetables is very important to your overall health and weight loss goals.

Foods that you should eat

Meats: You are free to choose any kind of meat including poultry, pork, beef, and lamb. You can even eat the skin on the chicken! Just make sure that when you prepare it, you're roasting it, frying it, broiling it, or grilling it without any breading or coating.

Shellfish and fish: You can eat any kind, but stick to the fattier kinds, such as mackerel, salmon, herring, and sardines.

Fats: Saturated and monounsaturated fats in egg yolks, avocados, macadamia nuts, coconut oil, olive oil, and butter are encouraged.

Eggs: You can cook eggs anyway you like, from fried, to boiled. They are an excellent source of protein.

Dairy: Make sure when you choose dairy products they are full-fat such as sour cream, butter, and full-fat cheeses.

Vegetables: Vegetables that are low in starch are encouraged on a low carb diet. These include lettuce, spinach, zucchini, broccoli, kale, artichokes, asparagus, brussels sprouts, bell peppers, avocados, olives, cucumbers, tomatoes, mushrooms, and onions.

Nuts: Choose nuts highest in protein and low in carbs, but these should be eaten in small amounts.

Foods to avoid

Sugar: This is a low-carb dieter's worst enemy. You'll find sugar in most juices, soft drinks, cookies, cakes, and cereals.

Starches: Breads, potatoes, pasta, chips, wheat, and rice.

Fruits: Fruits can be tricky when you're following a low carb diet because they are packed with natural sugars and carbohydrates. You want to avoid fruit that contains a lot of sugar. Even apples and bananas, which are often celebrated on weight loss diets, are to be avoided because of their sugar and carb content. The fruits lowest in carbs are blueberries, raspberries, and cantaloupe.

Processed Foods: Stay away from processed or packaged foods and hydrogenated fats like margarine. Chips, crackers, and even cans of soup or tomato sauce are often loaded with additional carbohydrates that you don't need.

In summary, a low-carb diet is a way of life rather than just a diet to lose weight. The 39 delicious low carb recipes in this book will hopefully have you excited about eating well. You will notice a number of improvements in your health and your life. Enjoy the weight loss and the food that makes it easy.

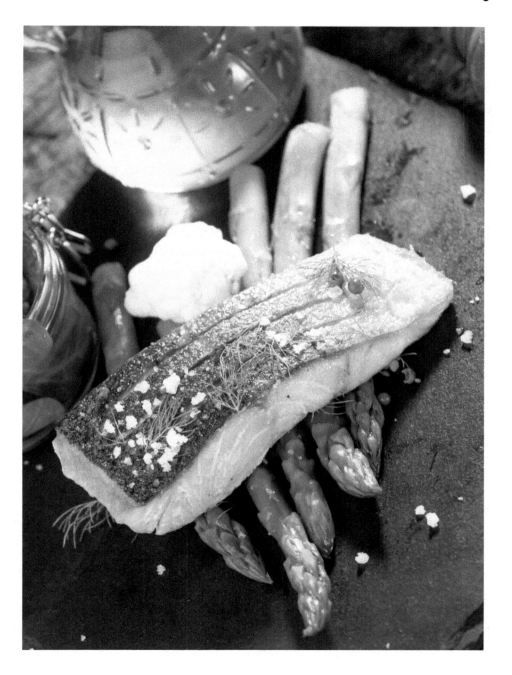

Chapter 2: Low Carb Salad Recipes

Salads are the cornerstone of any healthy eating plan, regardless of the one you choose. Low carb diets also embrace salads, and the beauty of these low carb salad recipes is that they combine a variety of vegetables with diverse sources of protein. You can also experiment with dressings; there are many different types of salad dressings and vinaigrettes that don't contain any carbohydrates, or have very low levels of carbs. Dressing them with olive oil and your favorite vinegar is a great way to introduce sharp, tangy flavors, and you can also be sure you're getting a fantastic helping of healthy fats from the oil. Remember to skip the croutons and anything containing sugar.

Steak and Cesar Salad

Yield: 6 servings
Ingredients:
1 pound romaine lettuce, chopped
1 pound grilled or broiled steak, sliced
½ cup parmesan cheese
1 cup olive oil
2 cloves garlic
2 anchovy filets
1 egg yolk
4 tablespoons red wine vinegar

Directions:
Toss the romaine, parmesan cheese and steak in a large salad bowl.

In a blender or mini chopper, puree the oil, vinegar, garlic, anchovies, and egg yolk. Pour over the salad and mix to combine.

Italian Antipasto Salad

Yield: 4 servings

Ingredients:

6 ounces mozzarella cheese, chopped

½ stick pepperoni, chopped

5 cups romaine lettuce, chopped

3 cups radicchio lettuce, chopped

½ cup marinated artichokes, chopped

½ cup mushrooms, chopped

1 stalk celery, chopped

½ red onion, sliced

1 cup grape tomatoes, chopped

¼ cup roasted red peppers, chopped

¼ cup olive oil

3 tablespoons balsamic vinegar

Directions:

Combine all the vegetables and top with the pepperoni and cheese.

Add the olive oil and the vinegar and toss together.

Low Carb Chicken Salad

Yield: 3 servings

Ingredients:

2 cups baby spinach
1 avocado, peeled and pitted
1 chicken breast
1 tablespoon Peri Peri Sauce
2 slices bacon

Directions:

1. Heat a pan over medium heat and cook the bacon until it is brown and crispy. Set the bacon aside.

2. Cut the chicken breast into strips, put in the bacon fat, and let them cook for 1 minute on one side then turn on the other side and fry for about 5 minutes.

3. Slice the avocado and bacon into small pieces.

4. Put the avocado and spinach in a large bowl, add the chicken, bacon, and Peri Peri sauce.

5. Toss and serve.

Tuna Salad with Lettuce

Yield: 4 servings

Ingredients:

2 cans of tuna, drained
1 stalk celery, chopped
¼ red onion, chopped
1 teaspoon dried oregano
1 teaspoon dried basil
1 tablespoon mayonnaise
Salt and Pepper
8 cups whole leaf butter lettuce

Directions:

Lay the lettuce out on a plate. In a small bowl, mix the tuna, celery, onion, and spices.

Add the mayonnaise and salt and pepper and combine. Scoop the tuna salad onto the lettuce.

Cheeseburger Salad

Yield: 4 servings
Ingredients:
1 pound ground beef, cooked
½ cup shredded cheddar cheese
½ pound romaine lettuce, chopped
½ iceberg lettuce, chopped
2 tomatoes, chopped
½ red pepper, chopped
½ cup red onion, chopped
2 tablespoons spicy mustard
½ lemon, juiced

Directions:
Mix the lettuces with the tomatoes, peppers and onions and cover with lemon juice, then set aside.

Combine the hot ground beef with the shredded cheese and mustard. Pour the meat mixture on top of the salad and combine.

Add a low carb salad dressing if it tastes dry.

Tomato and Cucumber Salad with Chicken

Yield: 4 servings

Ingredients:

2 cucumbers, chopped

½ red onion, sliced

4 tomatoes, chopped

1 cup olives, sliced

2 cups cooked chicken

2 stalks celery, chopped

3 tablespoons olive oil

2 tablespoons balsamic vinegar

Fresh basil

Salt and pepper

Directions:

Combine the cucumbers, tomatoes, olives, chicken, onion, and celery.

Cover with olive oil and vinegar, sprinkle with salt and pepper and top with fresh basil.

Bacon and Egg Salad

Yield: 4 servings

Ingredients:

6 slices bacon, cooked and chopped

4 eggs, boiled and chopped

2 cups spinach leaves

2 cups romaine lettuce

2 cups red leaf lettuce

2 cups green leaf lettuce

¼ cup red onion, sliced

½ cup yellow bell pepper, chopped

½ cup sundried tomatoes

¼ cup olive oil

3 tablespoons red wine vinegar

Directions:

Combine all of the lettuces, spinach, and vegetables. Add the olive oil and vinegar and toss together.

Top with the eggs and the bacon.

Chinese Chicken Salad

Yield: 4 servings

Ingredients:
1 head Napa cabbage, chopped
1 pound cooked chicken, chopped
2 stalks celery, minced
1 red bell pepper, minced
½ cup green onions, minced
½ cup chopped fresh cilantro
¼ cup soy sauce
¼ cup white wine vinegar
3 tablespoons fresh ginger, grated
3 tablespoons olive oil
¼ cup slivered almonds

Directions:
Toss the cabbage, chicken, celery, pepper, and onions together.

In a small bowl, whisk the soy sauce, vinegar, ginger and olive oil until combined. Cover the salad with the dressing and toss.

Sprinkle with cilantro and almonds.

Pizza Salad

Yield: 4 servings

Ingredients:

4 tomatoes, chopped and seeded
1 green bell pepper, chopped
1 cup sliced pepperoni
4 ounces mozzarella cheese, cubed
4 ounces provolone cheese, cubed
¼ cup shaved parmesan cheese
6 cups arugula
¼ cup sliced red onions
½ cup mushrooms, sliced
¼ cup olive oil
3 tablespoons red wine vinegar
Salt and pepper

Directions:

Cover a plate or a platter with the arugula. Sprinkle with salt and pepper.

In a large bowl, combine the vegetables. Layer the veggies on top of the arugula and then place a layer of pepperoni and mozzarella and provolone cheeses on top of that.

Cover with olive oil and red wine vinegar. Top with the shaved parmesan.

Raw Veggie Salad with Egg

Yield: 2 servings

Ingredients:

3 hard-boiled eggs, peeled and sliced

2 cups broccoli, chopped

2 cups cauliflower, chopped

1 cucumber, chopped

1 bell pepper, chopped

½ cup mushrooms, chopped

½ cup olives, chopped

¼ cup ranch dressing

Directions:

Instead of tossing the salad, create layers on your plate. Start with the eggs, then create a column of broccoli, cauliflower, cucumber, peppers, and mushrooms.

Top with the olives and either drizzle the entire plate with ranch dressing or use it as a dipping sauce for the veggies.

Spinach and Shrimp Salad

Yield: 4 servings

Ingredients:

10 cups baby spinach
1 pound cooked shrimp
2 boiled eggs, crumbled
½ red onion, sliced
1 cup cooked bacon, chopped
2 tablespoons olive oil
3 tablespoons red wine vinegar
1 teaspoon spicy mustard
Salt and pepper

Directions:

Place the spinach into a large bowl and toss with shrimp, egg, onion, and bacon.

Whisk together olive oil, vinegar, mustard, salt, and pepper. Dress the salad and toss together.

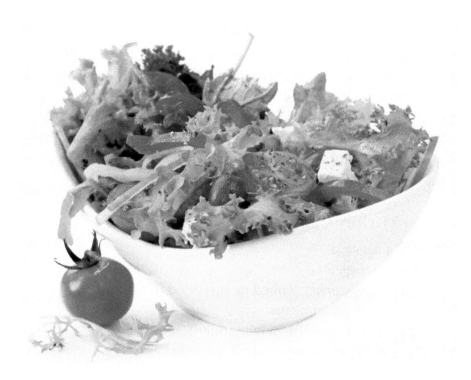

Chapter 3: Low Carb Oven Recipes

One of the best and easiest ways to cook good food is to throw your meal into the oven and leave it alone. When you're eating low carb, most of your food choices will involve meats and fish as well as vegetables. That means you have a lot of options when it comes to preparing hot, fresh meals that are healthy and full of protein, good fats, and all the things that are good for you. Try these low carb oven recipes. They're filling, fast, and fabulous.

Tomato Turkey Casserole

Yield: 4 servings
Ingredients:
2 cups cooked turkey, cubed or shredded
2 cups frozen green beans
2 cups tomato sauce (no sugar added)
3 tablespoons butter, separated
1 cup shredded cheddar cheese
¼ cup parmesan cheese

Directions:
Heat oven to 375 degrees F.

Mix turkey, green beans, and tomato sauce in a bowl to combine. Then, pour into a baking dish or a casserole dish. Cover with the cheddar and parmesan cheese.

Place 1 tablespoon of butter in 3 different places across the casserole. Cook for 30 minutes, until bubbling and brown.

Salmon and Squash

Yield: 4 servings

Ingredients:

2 green zucchini, sliced

2 yellow squash, sliced

¼ cup green onions

1 pound salmon fillet

2 tablespoons butter

¼ cup olive oil

1 teaspoon dried tarragon

Salt and pepper

Directions:

Preheat the oven to 400 degrees F. Grease a baking pan with butter and arrange the sliced zucchini and squash along the bottom. Add salt and pepper.

Place salmon fillet on top of the vegetables and cover with olive oil, green onions, and tarragon.

Bake for 30 minutes, until the salmon flakes easily.

Sausage and Eggplant Parmesan

Yield: 4 servings

Ingredients:

2 tablespoons olive oil

4 sausage links

2 small eggplants

2 cups crushed tomatoes

1 large egg

1 tablespoon heavy whipping cream

1 cup grated Parmesan cheese

2 cups shredded mozzarella cheese

1 tablespoon dried Italian herbs

Salt and pepper to taste

Fresh basil leaves

Directions:

1. Preheat oven to 350 degrees F, and heat the oil in a large skillet. Cook the sausage until brown and cooked through for about 12–15 minutes.

2. Slice the eggplant widthwise, and sprinkle with salt and pepper.

3. Remove sausage from skillet, leaving the oil and juices.

4. Mix the egg and cream together in one bowl and the Parmesan cheese and herbs in another bowl.

5. Dip each eggplant piece in the egg and then the Parmesan cheese. Fry in the skillet for 2 minutes on each side; remove to a casserole dish.

6. Cover each layer of eggplant with crushed tomatoes and mozzarella cheese, and place the sausages along the sides.

7. Bake for 20 minutes, and sprinkle with basil.

Bacon Shrimp

Yield: 4 servings

Ingredients:

1 pound shrimp, peeled and deveined

½ pound bacon strips, cut in half

1 tablespoon olive oil

2 tablespoons black pepper

Directions:

Preheat your oven to 400 degrees F. Wrap each shrimp with half a slice of bacon. Tuck the bacon under the shrimp or secure with a toothpick.

Spread the oil on a large baking sheet. Arrange all the shrimp on the baking sheet and sprinkle with pepper.

Cook for 15 minutes, until the bacon is crispy and the shrimp is pink. This dish goes well with spinach or even on top of a salad.

Chicken with Mushrooms

Yield: 4 servings
Ingredients:
4 chicken breasts
5 fresh white mushrooms, cut in half
5 fresh brown mushrooms (Crimini), cut in half
5 Shiitake mushrooms, cut in half
2 sprigs fresh rosemary
1 lemon, juiced
3 tablespoons olive oil
Salt and pepper

Directions:
Preheat oven to 350 degrees F.

Rub the chicken breasts with olive oil and place in a baking dish. Top with the selection of mushrooms and season with salt and pepper as well as the fresh rosemary.

Squeeze the lemon juice over the mushrooms and bake for 45 minutes.

Stuffed Peppers

Yield: 2 servings

Ingredients:
2 large bell peppers, sliced in half lengthwise
1 pound ground beef, cooked
½ cup parmesan cheese
¼ cup red onion, chopped
2 garlic cloves, minced
2 tomatoes, seeded and chopped
4 tablespoons tomato sauce
Salt and pepper

Directions:
Preheat the oven to 375 degrees F.

Place the peppers, skin side down in a baking dish. Fill each pepper with ground beef and then top with onion, garlic, tomatoes, and cheese. Cover with tomato sauce and season with salt and pepper.

Bake peppers in the oven for 30 minutes.

Citrus Chicken

Yield: 6–8 servings

Ingredients:

1 roasting chicken
1 lemon, sliced
1 lime, sliced
1 orange, sliced
4 cloves garlic
1 onion, sliced
3 stalks celery, cut in half
1 teaspoon dried oregano
1 teaspoon dried basil
1 teaspoon dried thyme
Salt and pepper
¼ cup olive oil

Directions:

Preheat oven to 350 degrees F. Layer the bottom of a baking dish with the onions, celery, and garlic.

Take the slices of lemon, lime and orange and gently insert them between the chicken skin and meat. The slices that won't fit can be placed in the chicken's cavity. Place the chicken on top of the vegetables and cover with olive oil and spices.

Bake for 1.5 hours or until a meat thermometer registers the chicken at 160 degrees.

Garlic Pork

Yield: 4 servings

Ingredients:

4 pork chops

2 eggs, beaten

2 tablespoons butter, melted

4 garlic cloves, smashed and minced

2 teaspoons salt

1 teaspoon cayenne pepper

2 teaspoons black pepper

1 pound fresh green beans, ends trimmed

2 tomatoes, sliced

2 tablespoons olive oil

Directions:

Preheat oven to 375 degrees F. Mix green beans and tomatoes in a bowl with olive oil.

Pour butter into a baking dish so the bottom is coated. Add the green beans and tomatoes.

Dip the pork chops in the egg. Place pork chops on top of the veggies and cover with smashed garlic, salt, and cayenne pepper.

Cook for 40 minutes.

Pepperoni Pizza

Yield: 6 servings
Ingredients:
For Crust:
2 cups mozzarella cheese
1 large egg
3 tablespoons cream cheese, softened
¾ cup almond flour
1 tablespoon psyllium husk
1 tablespoon Italian seasoning
Salt and pepper to taste
1 teaspoon butter, melted
For Topping
½ cup tomato sauce, no sugar added
16 pepperoni slices
1 cup mozzarella cheese, shredded
¼ teaspoon dried oregano, crushed

Directions:
1. Preheat oven to 400 degrees F.
2. For crust, in a microwave-safe bowl, place mozzarella cheese, and microwave on high for about 90 seconds or until melted completely.
3. Add eggs and cream cheese, and mix until well combined. Add remaining ingredients, and mix until well combined.
4. Coat the dough ball with melted butter, and place onto a smooth surface. With your hands, press the ball into a circular pattern.
5. Arrange the crust onto a baking sheet, and bake for about 10 minutes.
6. Carefully flip the side, and bake for about 2–4 minutes.
7. Remove the crust from oven. Spread the tomato sauce over crust.

8. Arrange the pepperoni slices evenly over tomato sauce, and sprinkle with cheese.

9. Bake for about 3–5 minutes. Remove from oven, and sprinkle with oregano.

10. Set aside to cool slightly. Cut into 6 wedges of equal size and serve.

Roasted Veggies and Sausage

Yield: 4 servings

Ingredients:

4 sausage links, sliced lengthwise

1 cup eggplant, peeled and chopped

1 cup zucchini, chopped

1 cup red onion, sliced

1 cup celery, chopped

¼ cup olive oil, plus extra for drizzling

1 teaspoon oregano

1 teaspoon basil

1 teaspoon rosemary

1 teaspoon red pepper flakes

Directions:

Preheat the oven to 375 degrees F. Drizzle a little olive oil on the bottom of a baking dish and place the sausages on the bottom of the pan, with the rounded side facing up.

In a bowl, combine the vegetables with the ¼ cup olive oil and the spices. Mix until all the veggies are coated.

Cover the sausages with the veggies. Cook for 40 minutes.

Cauliflower and Cheese

Yield: 4 servings

Ingredients:

1 head of cauliflower, chopped
6 slices of cooked bacon, chopped
½ cup sour cream
¼ cup green onions, sliced
½ cup parmesan cheese
¼ cup olive oil
Salt and pepper
1 cup shredded cheddar cheese

Directions:

Preheat the oven to 375 degrees F. Coat the bottom of a glass casserole dish with olive oil.

Combine the cauliflower, bacon, sour cream, green onions, and parmesan cheese in a bowl until everything is mixed together. Season the mixture with salt and pepper.

Spoon the mixture into the baking dish and flatten with the back of a spoon.

Add the shredded cheese to the top of the casserole and bake for 30 minutes, until everything is bubbling and brown.

Pumpkin Custard

Yield: 6 servings
Ingredients:
15 ounces pumpkin puree
4 eggs, beaten
½ cup heavy cream
2 teaspoons pumpkin pie spice
2 teaspoons vanilla extract
½ teaspoon liquid stevia
½ teaspoon salt
1/3 cup whipped cream

Directions:
1. Preheat oven to 350 degrees F. Grease 6 ramekins.
2. In a large bowl, add all ingredients except whipped cream, and beat until smooth.
3. Divide mixture evenly in prepared ramekins.
4. Bake for about 45–50 minutes or until a toothpick inserted in the center comes out clean.
5. Remove from oven, and place on a wire rack to cool.
6. Serve warm or cold with a topping of whipped cream.

Low Carb Meatloaf

Yield: 6 servings

Ingredients:

2 pounds ground beef

8 ounces tomato sauce (no added sugar)

¼ cup minced onion

3 garlic cloves, minced

2 eggs

3 tablespoons brown mustard

½ cup fine parmesan cheese

1 teaspoon salt

2 teaspoons pepper

Directions:

Preheat oven to 350 degrees F. Mix everything in the bowl, using your hands so it all gets mashed together.

Roll the meat into a loaf formation and place it in a roasting pan. Bake in the oven for 1 hour.

Take it out and let it rest for 15 minutes before eating.

Coconut Candy

Yield: 8 servings
Preparation Time: 5 minutes
Cooking Time: 50 minutes
Total Time: 55 minutes
Ingredients:
1 cup coconut oil, soft but not melted
4 tablespoons unsweetened cocoa powder
2 tablespoons almond butter
½ teaspoon liquid stevia
1 teaspoon vanilla extract
1 teaspoon sea salt

Directions:
1. Combine all ingredients in a bowl, and mix together with a spatula or your hands.

2. Once everything is combined, roll into balls, and place on a cookie sheet lined with foil.

3. Refrigerate for 30–40 minutes before serving.

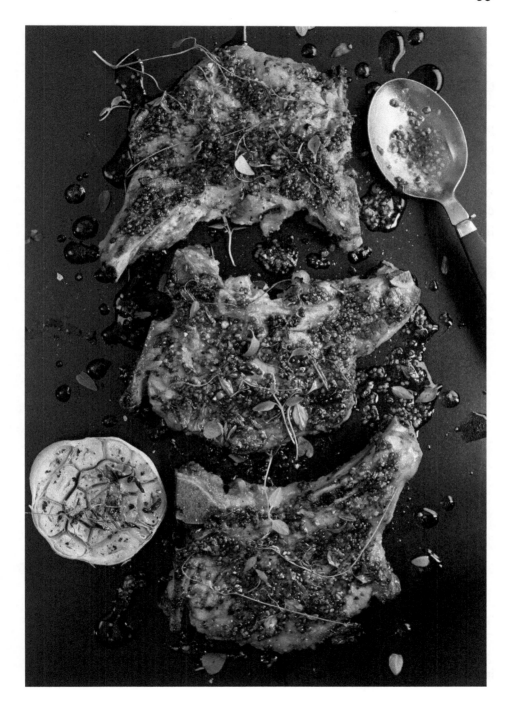

Chapter 4: Low Carb Slow Cooker Recipes

Cooking low carb meals that are healthy and packed with protein doesn't have to be time consuming or complicated. Slow cookers provide a great platform for preparing steaming hot food that doesn't require too much of your time and attention. You can toss everything into the pot, set the heat at the right level, and then go about your day while your nourishing and healthy meal cooks itself. Try these low carb slow cooker recipes and see how easy it is to live a low carb lifestyle.

Pesto Chicken

Yield: 3 servings
Ingredients:
2 cups spinach, chopped
1 cup fresh basil leaves, chopped
½ cup walnuts
2 tablespoons olive oil
½ lemon, juiced
1 tablespoon parmesan cheese
¼ cup pine nuts
1 pound cooked chicken, shredded or cubed
2 garlic cloves
½ white onion, sliced
½ cup sundried tomatoes
1 cup chicken broth
Salt and pepper

Directions:
In a small bowl, mix the spinach, basil, walnuts, olive oil and lemon juice until it has a paste-like texture.

Place the chicken in your slow cooker and cover with the pesto mix you just prepared. Then, add the cheese, pine nuts, garlic, onion, and tomatoes.

Season with salt and pepper and then cover with the chicken broth. Cook on low for 4 hours.

Breakfast Casserole

Yield: 6 servings
Ingredients:
8 eggs, beaten
1 sweet potato, chopped
1 pound breakfast sausage, chopped
1 red onion, sliced
2 cloves garlic, minced
1 red bell pepper, chopped
1 zucchini, chopped
Salt and pepper

Directions:
Put all the ingredients into a crock pot and mix well. Sprinkle with salt and pepper. Cook on low for six hours.

The casserole will set so that you can slice it like a pie or a cake—into squares or wedges.

Bacon and Veggie Omelet

Yield: 6 servings

Ingredients:

12 ounces frozen spinach, drained and thawed

6 slices bacon

12 eggs, lightly beaten

1 tablespoon olive oil

2 cups chopped mushrooms

1 cup red bell pepper, chopped

2 cups cream

½ teaspoon black pepper

¼ teaspoon salt

Directions:

1. Cook bacon in a skillet until crisp. Crumble and set aside.

2. In the bacon drippings, cook mushrooms and peppers until they are soft.

3. Add spinach and olive oil and cook for one more minute.

4. In a bowl, combine the eggs and cream, stir in the salt and pepper. Add the eggs to the skillet just to warm them; you don't have to fully cook the eggs.

5. Put the egg mixture into the slow cooker and top with bacon. Cook on low for 4 hours or high for 2 hours.

Broccoli Chop Breakfast

Yield: 6 servings

Ingredients:

1 head of broccoli, chopped

12 ounces breakfast sausage, chopped

10 eggs

½ cup water

2 cloves garlic, sliced

Salt and pepper to taste

Directions:

1. Cook sausage in a skillet until brown.

2. Place half the broccoli on the bottom of your slow cooker. Put half the sausage on top of the broccoli and then add the rest of the broccoli and then the sausage, so it's layered.

3. In a bowl, whisk together the eggs, garlic, water, salt, and pepper until combined and pour over the ingredients in the slow cooker.

4. Cook on high for 2 hours or low for 4 hours.

Italian Meatballs

Yield: 4 servings
Ingredients:
1 pound ground beef
½ onion, chopped
1 celery stalk, minced
¼ cup parmesan cheese
1 egg
1 teaspoon dried basil
1 teaspoon dried oregano
Salt and pepper
4 tomatoes, chopped
1 can (14 ounces) stewed tomatoes

Directions:
Make the meatballs by combining beef, onion, celery, cheese, egg, basil, oregano, salt, and pepper. Roll into balls and place on a plate.

Pour the stewed tomatoes and fresh tomatoes into the slow cooker and place meatballs on top.

Cook for 6 hours on low heat.

Seafood Stew

Yield: 6 servings

Ingredients:

1 pound tilapia
1 pound medium shrimp, shelled and deveined
6 ounces chopped clams, with liquid
1 cup chopped onion
1 cup chopped celery
1 cup sliced mushrooms
3 garlic cloves, minced
15 ounces diced tomatoes
8 ounces clam juice
6 ounces tomato paste
½ cup water
1 tablespoon red wine vinegar
1 tablespoon olive oil
2 teaspoons dried oregano
2 teaspoons dried parsley
2 teaspoons dried basil
1 teaspoon red pepper flakes

Directions:

Place everything except the fish, shrimp and clams into the slow cooker and mix to combine. Cook on high for 4 hours.

Stir the fish, shrimp and clams into the stew and set the heat to low. Cook for 1 more hour.

Cabbage and Ribs

Yield: 3 servings

Ingredients:

3 pounds beef short ribs (about 6 ribs)

1 head of green cabbage, quartered

4 green onions, sliced

½ cup soy sauce

½ cup red wine vinegar

2 cloves garlic, minced

1 tablespoon fresh ginger, grated

½ teaspoon red pepper flaks

1 tablespoon sesame oil

Directions:

Combine all ingredients in a slow cooker with the cabbage on top.

Cook on low for 8 hours, until the meat on the ribs easily pulls away from the bone.

Spicy Beef Brisket

Yield: 12 servings

Ingredients:

1 tablespoon olive oil

1 large white onion, sliced

3 garlic cloves, minced

1 beef brisket (4 pounds)

½ teaspoon red pepper flakes, crushed

½ teaspoon paprika

½ teaspoon ground cumin

¼ teaspoon ground cinnamon

Salt and pepper to taste

½ cup beef broth

Directions:

1. Combine all ingredients in the slow cooker, and mix well.

2. Cook on low for 6 hours.

3. Uncover the slow cooker, and transfer the brisket onto a cutting board. Set aside for about 10 minutes before slicing.

4. With a sharp knife, cut into desired slices.

5. Serve with fresh green salad.

Lemon Pepper Cod with Asparagus

Yield: 4 servings

Ingredients:

4 fresh cod filets

1 bundle of asparagus

2 lemons

4 teaspoons black pepper, divided

4 teaspoons white pepper, divided

4 tablespoons butter, divided.

Directions:

Place each fish filet on a piece of foil. Cover with asparagus. Sprinkle with peppers and then squeeze the juice from half a lemon onto each fish filet.

Add 1 tablespoon of butter to each piece of fish and then wrap the foil around the fish until it is completely sealed.

Place the 4 packets in the slow cooker. Cook in the slow cooker on high for 2 hours.

Sausage and Peppers

Yield: 4 servings

Ingredients:

1 pound Italian sausage, sweet and hot
2 red bell peppers, chopped
2 green bell peppers, chopped
1 red onion, sliced
3 garlic cloves, chopped
1 tablespoon olive oil

Directions:

Heat the oil in a skillet and brown the sausage for about 10 minutes in the skillet.

Add it to the slow cooker and cover with peppers, onions, and garlic.

Cook on low for 5–6 hours.

Garlic Mushrooms

Yield: 3 servings

Ingredients:

1 pound white button mushrooms, quartered
3 garlic cloves, minced
¼ cup fresh parsley, chopped
Salt and pepper to taste
2 tablespoons butter, melted
1 teaspoon fresh lemon zest, grated finely

Directions:

1. Combine all ingredients in the slow cooker except lemon zest and butter, and mix well.

2. Set the slow cooker on high. Cover and cook for 2 hours.

3. Uncover the cooker, and drizzle with the melted butter.

4. Serve with a topping of lemon zest.

Balsamic Chicken

Yield: 4 servings

Ingredients:

4 chicken breasts

½ cup balsamic vinegar

1 red onion, sliced

2 garlic cloves, chopped

4 tablespoons spicy mustard

1 pound fresh green beans, stems and ends trimmed

2 tablespoons olive oil

Salt and pepper

Directions:

Coat each chicken breast with the mustard. Pour the olive oil into the slow cooker and place the chicken on top of it.

Add the onion, garlic, salt, and pepper. Add the green beans and pour the balsamic vinegar on top of everything. Cook on high for 4 hours.

Paprika Flavored Pork

Yield: 4 servings

Ingredients:

2 pounds pork tenderloin

1 cup chicken stock

½ cup chopped tomatoes

1 lime, juiced

1 tablespoon fresh cilantro

¼ cup chopped red onion

2 tablespoons smoked paprika

1 tablespoon olive oil

Salt and pepper

Directions:

Coat the bottom of the slow cooker with olive oil. Place the pork on top of the oil. Season with salt and pepper.

In a small bowl, combine the chicken stock, tomatoes, lime juice, cilantro, onion and paprika. Mix together and pour the mixture over the pork.

Cook on high for 4 hours.

Turkey Chili

Yield: 6 servings

Ingredients:

1½ pounds ground turkey breast

1 medium red onion, chopped

2 cloves garlic, chopped

1 celery stalk, chopped

½ jalapeno, diced

4 ounces tomato paste

6 tomatoes, chopped and seeded

12 ounces stewed tomatoes

2 tablespoons chili powder

1 tablespoon cayenne pepper

1 tablespoon red pepper flakes

1 bay leaf

Directions:

In a skillet, heat the ground turkey until it's cooked. Then, put it in the slow cooker and cover with onion, garlic, celery, and jalapeno.

Add the tomato paste and stir. Then, add the tomatoes, stewed tomatoes, and spices. Stir again until all ingredients are mixed.

Cook on low for 6–8 hours.

Conclusion

Eating a low carb diet is a great idea for weight loss and improving your health. As with any plan, the first few weeks are the toughest. However, once you get through the initial stage, restricting carbs becomes second nature. Best of all, you'll begin to look and feel your absolute best!

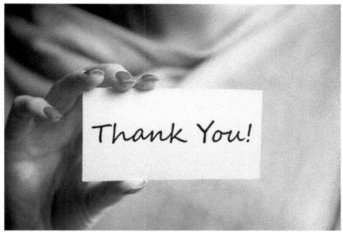

Finally, I want to thank you for reading my book. If you enjoyed the book, please take the time to share your thoughts and post a review on the book retailer's website. It would be greatly appreciated!

Best wishes,

Amanda Hopkins

Check Out My Other Books

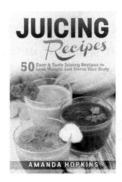

Juicing Recipes: 50 Easy & Tasty Juicing Recipes to Lose Weight and Detox Your Body

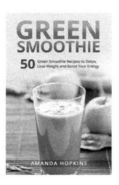

Green Smoothie: 50 Green Smoothie Recipes to Detox, Lose Weight and Boost Your Energy

Lightning Source UK Ltd.
Milton Keynes UK
UKHW022206060820
367821UK00004B/173